FGF21 - DIET: A 'MIRACLE HORMONE' THAT MAKES YOU SLIM?

A NEW APPROACH TO REPAIR YOUR METABOLISM AND GET SLIM?

MARCUS D. ADAMS

ISBN 978-1-63920-216-4

Contents

Preface

New research from the University of Sydney's Charles Perkins Centre suggests a low protein; high carbohydrate diet may be the most effective for stimulating a hormone with life-extending and obesity-fighting benefits.

The findings, paint a clearer picture of the role of a little-known hormone called Fibroblast Growth Factor 21 (FGF21) – the so-called 'fountain of youth' hormone produced primarily in the liver.

Previous studies have shown that FGF21 plays a role in curbing appetite, moderating metabolism, improving the immune system and extending lifespan. It is also currently being used as a therapeutic target for diabetes, though little is known about how this hormone is triggered and released in the body.

"Despite the popularity of high protein 'Paleo' diets, research suggests the exact opposite may be best for us as we age – that a low protein, high carbohydrate diet was the most beneficial for late life health and longevity,".

"The nutritional context in which FGF21 is most elevated is dependent on the balance of protein to carbohydrate, and this balance was also shown to be important in how this hormone helps to mediate protein hunger.

"These findings take us one step closer to understanding how FGF21 works, and as an extension of that to be able to use FGF21 to help people live longer and healthier lives."

"FGF21 has been shown to be elevated in really paradoxical conditions: in starvation and obesity, in cases of both insulin resistance and sensitivity and when there's a high and a low intake of food,"

"It appears that FGF21 is really switched on by a low protein intake, and its metabolic effects vary on whether it's coupled with high energy or low energy.

"Discovering more about how FGF21 is activated opens the way for nutritional interventions to chronic health problems, including as a potential drug target for the treatment of diabetes and other metabolic disorders. The next step will be to identify FGF21's exact signaling pathway in order to better tailor our diets and nutritional guidelines to generate the maximum benefit from this essential hormone."

ONE

THE MIRACLE HORMONE

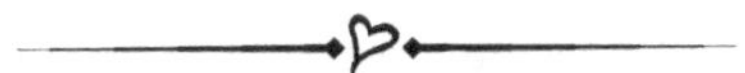

"There's been a lot of interest in this hormone called Fibroblast Growth Factor 21, and we know this can be influenced by diet. In fact, the hormone is now being called a miracle hormone or a 'fountain of youth' hormone.

"The reason why FGF21 is so interesting is because high levels of this hormone has been shown to play a huge role in driving things like appetite, improving metabolic health and immunity, and can even extend lifespan in mice."

If you're thinking 'yeah, in mice, not people', same results have been found in humans. It was also found that, again, a low-protein and high-carbohydrate diet rapidly increases FGF21 in the same way that it does in mice. Our findings are really possible to be translatable to humans,".

This particular diet has also been associated with improved markers of health -- for example, improved blood pressure, insulin levels, glucose levels, blood lipid levels and all these beneficial effects.

One of the most interesting parts about FGF21 is that the hormone can be elevated in "really conflicting conditions".

"For example, it can be elevated in starvation and obesity, or in high intake or low intake of food, or even in both insulin resistance and insulin team was able sensitivity,".

"Using nutritional framework, we took a look at all the data and looked at how macronutrients (proteins, carbohydrates and fats), as well as energy, interact together to influence levels of FGF21."Our research shows that a diet low in protein and high in carbohydrates was the most effective way to increase the levels of this hormone.

"This particular diet has also been associated with improved markers of health -- for example, improved blood pressure, insulin levels, glucose levels, blood lipid levels and all these beneficial effects."It makes it a very interesting hormone and, in fact, it's now being investigated as a therapeutic target for the treatment of cardiovascular disease and diabetes."

Now, you may be wondering what this ratio of carbs to protein is. Well, it's higher than you thought."We found that the optimum combination of protein and carbohydrates was one protein for 10 carbohydrates. So, a one in 10 ratio,"

"This is interesting because it seems to coincide beautifully with the diet of the Okinawan people of Japan, who are actually the longest lived population in the world. It's called the Okinawan diet."

Naturally the Okinawan people eat a low protein, high carbohydrate diet. If you're having a 'hallelujah' moment and are about to inhale all the cakes and doughnuts you possibly can, hold up.

"It's mainly lean meats and fish, and their carbohydrates are more of the complex, slowly digested carbohydrates, so your vegetables and high fibre foods. Not our current carbohydrates which are so easily accessible -- chips, doughnuts, pizza and pasta.

"So there's a clear distinction to be made that a low-protein, high-carbohydrate diet doesn't mean you can eat all the cake in the world."Yeah, not these kind of carbs unfortunately. In regards to the third macronutrient, fat, it doesn't have as much of an effect on FGF21 levels as carbohydrates.

"Fat didn't appear to have, in our mice at least, a major effect on driving FGF21 levels,".

"There is literature out there saying that a ketogenic diet increases it (a ketogenic diet means a high fat diet). However, when we look at it further, the reason why it increases, we think, is because it's a high-fat and low-protein diet, and that the low protein is the key to the elevation of FGF21."

If you're about to tell all your Paleo friends to suck it, don't be too hasty.

"I think there is something to be said for the high-protein diet in that it does help you lose weight.".Do not fear the delicious carb. However, that doesn't mean you have to choose between a super ripped body or eating lots of carbs (and possibly reduce your risk of lifestyle diseases and lengthen your life). You can do both.

"Exactly. It doesn't mean we have to stick with the same nutrient combination or diet throughout life. We can change it as we go, I think," I have no definitive evidence to say that, but I think eating a high protein diet when you're younger, and switching over to a lower protein diet could actually be beneficial to you."

Eating a protein restricted, high carbohydrate diet maximises FGF21, but this results in an increased appetite for protein, for which FGF21 may be responsible.

If FGF21 was the Fountain of Youth, then, to exploit this, you would need to eat in such a way that you would always be craving protein, and then, if you did eat enough protein, you'd lose your FGF21 advantage.

This does not sound like much fun, even for a mouse. Protein foods are flavorsome, come in considerable variety, and are excellent sources of vitamins, minerals, essential fats, and energy.

The LCHF diet isn't, and the Paleo diet needn't be high protein at all, but for humans there is a real advantage to keeping muscle on our bodies (mice, for example, don't need to open jars or lift the furniture often).

This helps us to stay active, makes us more useful in our daily lives, and helps with physical and mental health. Losing muscle because of some fad diet idea (sic) that involves restricting protein for longevity (rather than for some measurable shorter term benefit, which you can actually check) is perhaps not the first thing that scientists should promote in the media.

Surely every mouse experiment doesn't have to generate a headline – there are enough human experiments to be going on with. But I guess "high carbs key to long life" in a headline is just irresistible. The facts are, that all traditional, pre-industrial diets are more-or-less healthy except when resources are poor.

Populations eating diets high in meat and cheese (Sardinia) can be as long-lived as populations eating yams with low protein (Okinawa), and there are also shorter-lived populations eating both types of diet.

If we are no longer eating these traditional diets, we are more likely to have metabolic disease or other health conditions that are rare in traditional populations, and which usually respond to specific and perhaps novel dietary changes – even peasants emigrating from the Mediterranean 100 years ago were advised to stop eating carbohydrate foods if they became diabetic in their new homes.

Such changes can reasonably be expected to improve longevity for the individual more often than not.

Just in case you were avoiding all carbs like the plague, new research has suggested that a high carb, low protein diet is the most effective for stimulating a hormone with life-extending and obesity-fighting benefits.

The hormone in ?uestion is Fibroblast Growth Factor 21 also known as FGF21 if you're feeling particularly sciencey - which has been touted as the "fountain of youth" hormone.

TWO

METABOLIC ACTION OF FGF21

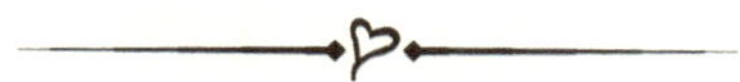

Fibroblast growth factor 21 (FGF21) is an atypical member of the FGF family that functions as an endocrine factor. In obese animals, elevation of plasma FGF21 levels by either pharmacological or genetic approaches reduces body weight, decreases hyperglycemia and hyperlipidemia, alleviates fatty liver and increases insulin sensitivity.

FGF21 exerts its pleiotropic metabolic effects through its actions on multiple targets, including adipose tissue, liver, brain and pancreas.

The expression of FGF21 is under the control of both peroxisome proliferator-activated receptor gamma (PPARγ) and peroxisome proliferator-activated receptor alpha (PPARα).

A growing body of evidence suggests that the metabolic benefits of these two nuclear receptors are mediated in part by induction of FGF21. In humans, plasma levels of FGF21 are elevated in obese subjects and patients with type 2 diabetes, but are reduced in patients with autoimmune diabetes.

This chapter summarizes recent advances in understanding the physiological roles of FGF21 and the molecular pathways underlying its actions, and also discusses the future prospective of developing FGF21 or its agonists as therapeutic agents for obesity-related medical complications.

Glucose and lipid metabolism is tightly controlled by a large number of metabolic hormones secreted from different endocrine organs.

Notable among them are the pancreatic hormones (insulin and glucagon), adipose tissue-secreted adipokines (such as leptin and adiponectin), gut-derived hormones (such as glucagon-like peptide-1 and ghrelin) and adrenal hormones (such as glucocorticoids).

These metabolic hormones form an integrated network to control substrate utilization and energy balance in response to nutritional status. Aberrant secretion and/or dysfunction of metabolic hormones are important contributor to obesity-related cardio-metabolic complications, including type 2 diabetes, nonalcoholic fatty liver disease, hypertension, coronary heart disease and stroke.

Several members of the fibroblast growth factors (FGFs) super family, including FGF15/19, FGF21 and FGF23, has recently been identified to play important roles in metabolic regulations4.

Unlike the classic FGFs that require heparin for stable binding to the FGF receptors (FGFRs), the three endocrine members of the FGF super family lack the heparin-binding property, and therefore can be released into the circulation to act as endocrine factors4.

These hormone-like FGFs are involved in the regulation of diverse metabolic pathways: FGF15/19 controls cholesterol/

bile acid synthesis, FGF23 modulates phosphate/vitamin D metabolism, and FGF21 regulates glucose and lipid metabolism.

Due to the multiple metabolic benefits of FGF21 on energy homeostasis and insulin sensitivity, it has attracted great attention as a potential therapeutic candidate for obesity-related medical complications.

Pharmacological effects of FGF21

The metabolic activity of FGF21 was first discovered by Kharitonenkov and colleagues in a cell-based high throughput screening as a positive hit for its ability to induce glucose uptake in adipocytes.

Therapeutic administration of recombinant FGF21 in both db/db diabetic mice and dietary obese mice lowers blood glucose and triglyceride levels, and also reverses hepatic steatosis and improves insulin sensitivity.

Transgenic mice with liver-specific overexpression of FGF21 are resistant to diet-induced obesity, possibly due to increased energy expenditure9. Likewise, chronic administration of FGF21 to diabetic rhesus monkey for a period of 6 weeks causes a dramatic decline in fasting levels of blood glucose, fructosamine, insulin and glucagon, and also improves lipid profiles, including lowering of triglycerides and low-density lipoprotein cholesterol and raising of high-density lipoprotein cholesterol6.

Notably, FGF21 does not induce mitogenicity and hypoglycemia at any dose tested in both rodents and rhesus monkeys demonstrating that FGF21 exhibits therapeutic characteristics necessary for effective treatment of diabetes and its complications.

However, it is of importance to note that therapeutic doses of recombinant FGF21 used for these studies are substantially higher than those in physiological concentrations.

It is currently unclear whether the re?uirement of supraphysiological doses for effective therapeutic intervention is due to the low bioactivity of recombinant FGF21 generated from E. coli, or due to FGF21 resistance in obese/diabetic animals.

Since FGF21 knockout (KO) mice do not develop either hyperglycemia or insulin resistance, it is also possible that the therapeutic benefits of recombinant FGF21 on glucose homeostasis are only of pharmacological interest, but not of physiological relevance

Metabolic actions of FGF21 on its major target tissues

HepaticFGF21 functions

The liver is a major site for both production and actions of FGF21.The hepatic expression and plasma levels of FGF21 in mice are markedly elevated upon fasting, but are suppressed by re-feeding.

Fasting-induced hepatic expression of FGF21 is mediated by PPARα, a ligand-activated transcriptional factor that plays a central role in controlling lipid metabolism and energy homeostasis.

The mRNA expression of FGF21 in both mouse livers and human primary hepatocytes are strongly induced by the PPARα agonists fenofibrates, whereas both fasting- and fenofibrates-induced expression of FGF21 is abrogated in PPARα KO mice.

A growing body of evidence suggests that FGF21 serves as a key downstream target of PPARα mediating the metabolic adaptation responses to fasting/starvation, including ketogenesis, fatty acid oxidation and gluconeogenesis.

FGF21 acts as a downstream target of PPARα exerting multiple biological effects ...

FGF21 acts as a downstream target of PPARα exerting multiple biological effects in hepatocytes. In response to fasting, free fatty acids (FFA) released from adipocytes acts as an endogenous ligand to activate PPARα, which induces FGF21 expression via transcriptional activation.

FGF21 released from hepatocytes may act in an endocrine or autocrine/paracrine manner modulating ketogenesis, gluconeogenesis, fatty acid oxidation, growth hormone (GH) resistance and carcinogenesis. Note that whether or not hepatocytes are a direct target of FGF21 is still a matter of debate.

Modulation of ketogenesisby FGF21

In response to fasting/starvation, hepatic metabolism is programmed to oxide fatty acids and to produce fuel in the form of ketone bodies (β-hydroxybutyrate, acetoacetate and acetone), which progressively becomes the major energy source for the brain 17. Several independent studies have demonstrated that FGF21 is re?uired for fasting-induced ketogenesis in mice.

Adenovirus-mediated in vivo knockdown of hepatic FGF21 expression in a ketogenic diet-fed mice causes fatty liver, lipemia, and reduced serum ketones, and this change is associated with altered expression of key genes involved in hepatic lipid metabolism and ketone production.

Vice versa, the transgenic mice with liver-specific overexpression of FGF21 exhibit a significant increase in serum concentrations of ketone bodies and a concurrent reduction in serum and hepatic triglyceride concentrations.

Furthermore, impaired ketone production (hypoketonemia) and hepatic steatosis in PPARα KO mice can be partially restored by administration of recombinant FGF21. However, two independent studies on FGF21 KO mice have yielded inconsistent data on the role of FGF21 in ketogenesis. FGF21 KO mice generated by Flier's group display impaired adaption to ketosis induced by a ketogenic diet, which is accompanied by severe hepatic steatosis and body weight gain as compared with wild type mice.

By contrast, Itoh and colleagues demonstrated a modest increase in serum β-hydroxybutyrate levels in FGF21 KO mice fasted for 24h, suggesting an increased ketogenesis. The differences in genetic background, diet composition and/or study protocols may account for the inconsistent observations between the two reports.

In humans, chronic treatments with the PPARα agonist fenofibrates increase the circulating concentrations of FGF21 19. However, ketogenic diet has no obvious influence on circulating FGF2120. The physiological roles of FGF21 in regulating ketogenesis need further investigation.

FGF21 and hepatic gluconeogenesis

PPARα is an important player in fasting-induced hepatic gluconeogenesis. PPARα KO mice exhibit hypoglycemia upon fasting, which is accompanied by impaired expression of gluconeogenic genes.

Likewise, FGF21 has been implicated in the regulation of gluconeogenesis during the progression from fasting to starvation. Such an effect of FGF21 is mediated by induction of hepatic expression of peroxisome proliferator-activated receptor coactivator protein 1 α (PGC1α), a transcriptional coactivator that controls the expression of gluconeogenic genes.

The inductive effects of FGF21 on expression of the two gluconeogenic genes (glucose-6-phosphatase and phosphoenolpyruvate carboxykinase) are virtually abrogated in PGC1α KO mice. Vice versa, mice lacking FGF21 fail to fully induce PGC1α expression in response to fasting and have impaired gluconeogenesis.

Notably, direct incubation of either isolated, perfused mouse liver or primary cultures of rat or mouse hepatocytes with FGF21 has no obvious effects on PGC1α expression, suggesting that FGF21 might stimulate gluconeogenesis through an indirect mechanism.

In contrast to the aforementioned findings, another study from Fisher and colleagues showed that FGF21 acts directly on the liver to stimulate the expression of gluconeogenic genes.

This study also found that FGF21 can still induce the same degree of gluconeogenic gene expression in mice with liver-specific ablation of PGC1α as seen in wild-type mice, thus excluding the involvement of PGC1α in FGF21-induced glucose production. The precise role of FGF21 on hepatic gluconeogenesis and the underlying mechanisms require further clarification.

FGF21 and fatty aid oxidation

PPARα is a master regulator of fatty acid oxidation, by inducing the expression of a cluster of key genes involved in this process.

A growing body of evidence suggests that induction of hepatic fatty acid oxidation by PPARα is mediated in part by FGF21. RNAi-mediated suppression of FGF21 expression causes impaired ketogenic diet-induced fatty acid oxidation and severe hepatic steatosis, whereas chronic treatment with recombinant FGF21 reverses fatty liver in diet-induced obese mice.

A recent study by Li and colleagues found that sodium butyrate, a dietary compound with protective effects against diet-induced obesity and dyslipidemia, increases hepatic expression and plasma levels of FGF21 in mice.

Noticeably, the ability of sodium butyrate to increase energy expenditure and fatty acid oxidation was abrogated in FGF21 KO mice. In humans, plasma levels of FGF21 are significantly elevated in patients with fatty liver disease and are positively correlated with the liver fat percentage and the degree of steatosis.

It is currently unclear whether elevated plasma FGF21 levels are due to the compensatory responses or the presence of FGF21 resistance to fatty acid oxidation.

THREE

FGF21 AND GROWTH HORMONE RESISTANCE

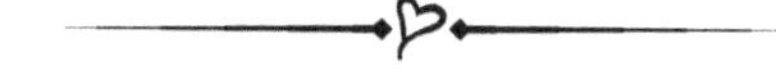

GH is synthesized and secreted by the anterior pituitary to regulate growth and metabolism. Many GH actions are mediated by induction of hepatic expression of insulin-like growth factor 1 (IGF-1).

Starvation is known to block the growth actions of GH by decreasing hepatic production of IGF-1 through mechanisms that are not well understood. In this connection, FGF21 has been proposed as a key mediator conferring the starvation-induced inhibition on the GH/IGF-1 axis, by suppression of the active form of signal transducer and activator of transcription 5 (STAT5), whereby leading to a reduction of IGF-1 expression.

Furthermore, FGF21 also induces the expression of IGF-1 binding protein-1 and suppressor of cytokine signaling, which further blunt GH signaling. Consistent with this report, FGF21 KO mice exhibit greater body and tibial growth than their wild-type littermates after 4 weeks of food restriction, whereas single injection of GH induces greater hepatic activation of STAT5 and induction of IGF-1 in FGF21 KO mice than in wild-type mice.

The suppressive effect of FGF21 on GH signaling is also supported by another finding showing that FGF21 serves as a negative feedback regulator to block GH-induced lipolysis in adipocytes.

Suppression of hepatic IGF-1 production by FGF21 may also explain the delayed onset of chemically-induced hepatocarcinogenesis; Consistent with these animal-based findings, plasma levels of FGF21 are significantly elevated in patients with anorexia nervosa, a state of chronic nutritional deprivation characterized by GH resistance with elevated GH levels and decreased levels of IGF-1.

In subjects with elevated FGF21 levels, there was a strong inverse association between FGF21 and IGF-1, suggesting that FGF21 may mediate GH resistance in humans.

FGF21 actions in adipose tissue

White adipocytes are another major target cells of FGF21, where it stimulates glucose uptake, modulates lipolysis, enhances mitochondrial oxidative capacity, and potentiates PPARγ activity. There is also good evidence that FGF21 is involved in the thermogenic functions of brown adipocytes.

Pleiotropic metabolic actions of FGF21 in adipocytes. FGF21 may act in an Pleioautocrine/paracrine manner to regulate glucose uptake, lipid metabolism and PPARγ activity in white adipocytes, and increases the thermogenic activity of brown adipocytes.

Stimulation of glucose uptake by FGF21

In both 3T3-L1 adipocytes and human primary adipocytes, FGF21 potently stimulates glucose uptake in an insulin-independent manner5. Unlike insulin, FGF21 has no effect on plasma membrane translocation of the glucose transporter GLUT4, but induces the expression of GLUT1 through transcriptional activation.

FGF21 stimulates mitogen-activated protein kinase or extracellular signal-regulated kinases (ERK1/2)], which in turn phosphorylates and activates the transcription factors serum response factor (SRF) and Ets-like protein-1 (Elk-1) in 3T3-L1 adipocytes.

Activated SRF and Elk-1 act synergistically to transactivate the GLUT1 gene by binding to the highly conserved serum response element and E-26 motifs within the promoter region. FGF21-induced phosphorylation of ERK1/2 and SRF/Elk1, GLUT1 expression and glucose uptake are blunted in adipose tissue of obese mice as compared to lean controls, suggesting the existence of FGF21 resistance in obesity.

However, whether or not FGF21-induced glucose uptake accounts for its glucose-lowering effects remains to be determined.

Regulation of lipolysis by FGF21

Conflicting data related to the roles of FGF21 on lipolysis has been reported. An early study in 3T3-L1 adipocytes demonstrated that acute treatment of recombinant FGF21 increases lipolysis.

By contrast, another report found that chronic treatment of 3T3-L1 adipocytes or human adipocytes with either murine or human FGF21 for a period of 3 day has no obvious effects on basal glycerol release, but leads to a marked attenuation in noradrenaline- and forskolin-induced lipolysis.

Likewise, a single injection of FGF21 acutely reduces plasma free fatty acid (FFA) levels similar to its acute effects on plasma glucose in db/db mice. In vitro, FGF21 also inhibits lipolysis in adipocytes during a short treatment and decreases total lipase activity.

The inhibitory effect of FGF21 on lipolysis is also confirmed by our recent study showing that FGF21 suppresses GH-induced lipolysis through a negative feedback regulatory loop.

In response to fasting/starvation, GH is released from the pituitary gland to stimulate lipolysis in adipocytes for the release of FFAs, which in turn induce hepatic FGF21 production via activation of PPARα. Elevated FGF21 in turn acts as a negative feedback signal to terminate GH-induced lipolysis in adipocytes.

Such a feedback regulation not only helps to maintain the balance of lipid distribution between liver and adipose tissue, but also prevents lipotoxicity caused by sustained elevation of FFAs.

These findings also suggest that the insulin-sensitizing effect of FGF21 may be attributed to its ability in inhibiting the excessive elevation of circulating FFA induced by the lipolytic hormones such as GH.

The suppressive effect of FGF21 on lipolysis during fasting is also supported by a recent report in FGF21 KO mice. However, this study also suggests that FGF21 may play an opposite role during the fed state.

In humans, the 24-h profiles of circulating FFAs closely resemble those of FGF21. There is a strong positive association between the peak concentrations of circulating FFAs and FGF21 during both the daytime and nighttime.

Noticeably, the peak time of circulating FFAs precedes that of FGF21 by approximately 3–4 h, matching well with the in vitro observation that incubation of human hepatocytes with fatty acids for this period induces the production of FGF21.This study also support the existence of a feedback regulation between FGF21 and FFAs may account for the circadian rhythm of both factors in humans.

Reciprocal regulation between FGF21 and PPARγ

Although the liver is the main contributor to circulate FGF21, data from both animals and humans suggest that adipocytes also express and secrete FGF21, which is under the control of PPARγ.

Notably, FGF21 expression in adipocytes is increased in the fed state and is decreased in the fasting state, a pattern opposite to that in hepatocytes. Furthermore, this study demonstrated the existence of a feed-forward loop between FGF21 and PPARγ in adipocytes, which may confer the insulin-sensitizing actions of the anti-diabetic drugs thiazolidinediones (TZDs).

FGF21 KO mice display defects in PPARγ signaling, including decreased body fat and reduced expression of PPARγ-dependent genes, and also resistant to both the beneficial insulin-sensitizing effects and the detrimental weight gain and edema side effects of the PPARγ agonist rosiglitazone.

Such a change in FGF21 KO mice is accompanied by a marked increase in the sumoylation of PPARγ, which blocks its transcriptional activity and possibly by promoting corepressor recruitment.

This unexpected finding suggests that FGF21 has two separate physiological functions: as an endocrine factor secreted by the liver to coordinate the adaptive response to fasting/starvation, and as an autocinre factor induced in WAT during the fed state to regulate adipocyte function.

FGF21 and thermogenesis in brown adipocytes

Brown adipose tissue (BAT) is the main site of non shivering thermogenesis in rodents and human neonates, and functional BAT may also exist in human adults. A growing body of evidence suggests FGF21 as an important thermogenic regulator through its autocrine functions in brown adipocytes.

FGF21 expression in brown adipocytes of mice is relatively high compared to white adipocytes, and is strongly induced by either cold challenge or β-adrenergic agonists through induction of cAMP and MAP kinase.

Notably, cold challenge increases circulating FGF21 without affecting hepatic FGF21 expression, suggesting that BAT becomes the major source of circulating FGF21 under this circumstance.

Injection of FGF21 into neonatal mice increases body temperature, enhances the expression of genes involved in thermogenesis and promotes uncoupling respiration within BAT. FGF21 is also implicated in the conversion of white adipocytes into a "brown-like" state.

FGF21 KO mice display an impaired ability to adapt to chronic cold exposure, with diminished browning of WAT. This effect of FGF21 may be attributed to its ability in enhancing PGC1α expression in adipose tissue. Indeed, FGF21 has been shown to activate AMP-activated protein kinase and SirT1, thereby leading to enhanced mitochondrial oxidation through activation of PGC1α in adipocytes.

In support of the role of FGF21 as a stimulator of thermogenesis in BAT, transgenic expression or therapeutic administration of FGF21 increases energy expenditure and decreases body weight in mice.

However, FGF21 KO mice exhibit a similar12 or even slightly decreased body weight and fat mass as compared to wild-type controls. The physiological functions of FGF21 in BAT need further investigation.

Central FGF21 actions

The brain plays a central role in controlling body fat content and glucose and lipid homeostasis. FGF21 can cross blood–brain barrier and enter the brain in a non-saturable manner50, and has been proposed as a missing link between the brain and the peripheral metabolic tissues.

Chronic intracerebroventricular infusion of recombinant FGF21 into the lateral cerebral ventricle increases food intake, energy expenditure, and hepatic insulin sensitivity in male obese rats, suggesting that the metabolic effects of FGF21 are mediated in part through its central actions.

FGF21 has also been proposed as a possible signal peptide to convey the information of PPARα activation from the liver to brain to induce "torpor", a state of decreased physiological activity in animals characterized by a reduced body temperature and metabolic rate as an adaptive response to conserve energy.

Administration of the PPARα agonist bezafibrate induces a time-dependent torpor-like phenomenon and concurrently increases hepatic FGF21 production in mice. Interestingly, both transgenic expression and therapeutic administration of FGF21 stimulate torpor in mice.

Likewise, intracerebroventricular injection of neuropeptide Y (NPY) also reliably induces torpor-like hypothermia that resembles natural torpor in hamsters. Since the PPARα agonist bezafibrate also stimulate NPY production, it has been suggested that PPARα controls torpor and circadian clock through the FGF21-NPY axis.

However, there is currently no evidence demonstrating that FGF21 acts as an upstream regulator of NPY.

Thepancreatic actionsof FGF21

Several independent studies on different animal models have consistently demonstrated the protective effects of FGF21 against various pancreatic injury as well as β-cell dysfunction. FGF21 KO mice are more susceptible to cerulein-induced pancreatitis (CIP), whereas FGF21 transgenic mice are resistant to develop this acute pancreatic damage.

The protection of FGF21 against CIP is possibly attributed to its ability in activation of ERK1/2 in pancreatic stellate cells. FGF21 expression can be detected in human, rat and mouse pancreatic islets as well as in rat primary β-cells and INS-1E cells.

Short-term administration of FGF21 lowers plasma insulin concentrations in both healthy and db/db mice, whereas long-term treatment with FGF21 increases both the number of islets and the amount of insulin per islet in db/db mice. However, FGF21 did not affect islet cell proliferation.

Treatment of rat islets or INS-1E cells causes a partial protection against glucotoxicity- and cytokine-induced apoptosis, possibly by activation of both ERK1/2 and Akt signaling pathways.

In addition, FGF21 suppresses glucagon secretion from isolated rat islets and reduces plasma glucagon concentrations in mice5. FGF21 also enhances islet engraftment in mouse synergetic islet transplantation model.

Transplantation of islets pre-treated with FGF21 for three days into streptozocin-induced diabetic mice restores normoglycemia by suppressing islet graft loss.

FOUR

THE MAGICAL HORMONE THAT MAKES YOU SLIM

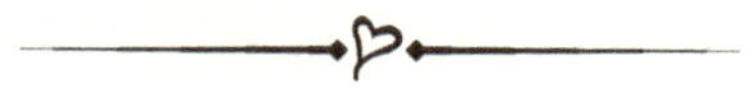

Since its initial discovery in 2000 by researchers in Japan, the hormone known as fibroblast growth factor-21 (FGF21) has intrigued biologists and endocrinologists. Mouse FGF21 is highly identical to human FGF21, making it useful for laboratory comparison.

It didn't take long for investigators to realize FGF21 is a "novel therapeutic agent for human metabolism" in the regulation of sugar utilization, particularly in fat cells (adipocytes) in the liver.

Therapeutic provision of FGF21 to laboratory mice reduces blood sugar levels and these animals are resistant to obesity. And FGF21 does not induce hypoglycemia (low blood sugar), cancer or weight gain at any tested dose in diabetic or healthy animals. Biologists were beginning to think of it as an ideal hormone/drug to treat diabetes.

The biological activity exhibited by FGF21 was found to be dependent upon a gene called Klotho that makes beta-klotho protein that in turn increases the ability of cell receptors for FGF21 to direct its beneficial effects upon fat cells in particular.

Researchers also discovered that FGF21 interplays with a metabolic pathway called PPAR (peroxisome proliferator-activated receptor) that aids in the transport of sugar to fat cells and the burning of fat.

Since an energy supply is essential for life to be maintained, researchers were elated to find that FGF21 helps to maintain energy in living cells during starvation or fasting. This makes FGF21 a necessary hormone to facilitate hibernation in animals since they obviously don't consume food during that time.

How it works

During periods of fasting, starvation or hibernation, cells must still produce energy or die. When food is withheld from animals for 12 hours or longer, liver cells produce FGF21. Researchers found that FGF21 switches the body to a fat-burning mode and allows the body to fuel itself with stored fat during times of food deprivation.

FGF21 mobilizes lipids from fat cells and directs the liver to transform those energy-rich molecules to circulate throughout the body. Just the provision of FGF21 by itself produces the same biological responses as fasting without having to deprive calories.

One researcher says FGF21 has "almost magical properties" as it improves insulin efficiency, lowers circulating levels of cholesterol and triglycerides and averts age-related weight gain.

Biologists were not only beginning to think FGF21 is a remedy for diabetes, but it could also prevent obesity after it was found that administration of FGF21 to laboratory mice resulted in a 20% reduction in weight.

A human population study finds that elevated blood serum levels of FGF21 are associated with abnormal blood sugar metabolism and insulin resistance seen among patients with metabolic disease (diabesity).

However, it should not be misconstrued that increased amounts of FGF21 induce metabolic disease. It just means this defensive hormone is increased as metabolism goes haywire.

Interest in FGF21 by drug companies ensued as pharmacologists began to make FGF21 look-alike molecules (analogs) in hopes of producing "superior metabolic" action. FGF21 could become the most advanced weapon against diet-induced diseases ever imagined.

FGF21- An anti-aging agent?

But then investigators gleefully found that FGF21 also inhibits growth hormone. That would also place FGF21 in a class of potential anti-aging molecules. Of interest, vitamin D increases Klotho protein to regulate calcium and phosphate in the body and thus also serves as an anti-aging agent. FGF21 re?uires klotho protein to function. Two known anti-aging agents were found to work in tandem.

These discoveries were very tantalizing for researchers. They didn't want to jump to conclusions. They needed a lifespan study. Laboratory mice live about 12-18 months.

So researchers at University of Texas Southwestern Medical Center in Dallas launched a study to determine if in fact FGF21 will prolong the life of laboratory mice.

Their efforts exceeded expectation. But their investigation also wiped the biological drawing board clean and forced biologists to re-think everything they have learned in the past decade.

Remarkably, genetically altering laboratory mice so they produce about 5-10 times more FGF2 during fasting resulted in a striking increase in lifespan without reducing food intake.

These super-mice lived about 36% longer than normal mice and astoundingly better than 30% of the female mice in the study were still alive at 44 months of age when the study was finalized. The risk of death was reduced by 65% in male animals, 88% in females.

These animals apparently burned away their fat much more efficiently. The revved-up FGF21 mice were leaner than normal mice even though they ate about the same amount of food.

Surprising pathway

But all this was accomplished without activating other well-known longevity pathways (sirtuin genes, AMP kinase, mTOR and NAD+). Unexpectedly, calorie restriction, known to double the lifespan of laboratory animals by cutting caloric intake in half, did not trigger FGF21 hormone production.

These genetically altered mice are smaller than normal mice as they produce less growth factor (insulin-like growth factor 1 or IGF1). While life-prolonging long-term calorie restriction significantly alters 831 genes in laboratory mice, FGF21-producing mice achieved super-longevity by altering only a small number of genes.

It first appeared humanity was on the cusp of a giant breakthrough that could promote health and prolong life beyond any prior imagined mechanism. But there was one drawback. These FGF21 super-mice developed weak bones. Bone loss in these animals "may limit its utility as a therapeutic agent" the researchers disappointingly disclose.

So what is the take-home message of this discovery? What can modern longevity-seeking humans do to activate

FGF21?

Fasting (breakfast skipping)

One life-prolonging practice might be to periodically fast. A 12-hour fast activates FGF21 which then begins to increase fat burning. There are some people who never eat breakfast, to prolong their daily fasting period.

While most dieticians say skipping breakfast leads to overeating and obesity, almost all of the studies on this topic have been performed among growing children. Children are growing, not aging, and certainly don't fit into the category of middle-agers who are experiencing mid-body weight gain.

A study of over 5800 men reveals that breakfast skipping modestly contributes to weight gain. A small study shows two-day a week fasting among adult males reduces weight.

Limitation of phosphorus

Another approach might be to limit phosphorus in the diet. That is because the aforementioned klotho protein limits excessive over-calcification and phosphorus in the human body.

To understand the relevance of phosphorus limitation to aging an understanding of the klotho gene is re?uired.

There is evidence that adults who have lower levels of klotho protein in their blood circulation have an increased risk of death. Since FGF21 requires klotho protein to work, investigation into mechanisms of klotho formation may be advantageous. Mice that are bred to produce more klotho protein live about 17.4% longer, not ?uite as striking as FGF21 itself, but still would add more than a decade to humans if animal research has application in humans.

In explaining how klotho works, researchers reveal that dietary phosphate restriction reverses aging in laboratory mice bred to not produce klotho protein. There is genetic and dietary evidence that phosphate toxicity accelerates aging. When mice are bred so as not to produce klotho protein and fed a high phosphate diet, signs of premature aging appear.

Researchers in Japan are concerned about increasing amounts of dietary phosphorus which may accelerate aging. Restriction of phosphorus and calcium is advised. House flies (Drosophila melanogaster), used in longevity experiments, age prematurely when provided with a high phosphorus diet.

Many fast foods have phosphate additives. Excessive phosphorus should be considered a health risk.

One of the confusing aspects of understanding phosphorus in the diet is that plant foods provide a natural calcium and phosphorus balancing agent called phytate (inositol hexaphosphate or IP6) provided in plant foods which inhibits the digestion of these minerals significantly (from ~80% to ~20%0.

It is the inorganic phosphorus in food additives, prevalent in fast foods, that is the culprit here. Supplemental IP6 is available as an extract from rice bran and should be considered a powerful anti-aging substance via its ability to calcifications and phosphorus overload.

Researchers in Japan report on a novel way to increase FGF21 hormone via inhalation of hydrogen gas or consumption of hydrogen-fortified drinking water. Mice given hydrogen water lost excessive weight experienced a decline in blood sugar, insulin and triglycerides, all which was correlated with an increase in FGF21.

For the really serious pursuers of longevity, on the commercial side there is even a hydrogen drinking water produced in Malaysia that is touted for its health benefits (though no evidence is provided this beverage has any health benefits).

Other ways to increase FGF21 would be to take the anti-diabetic drug metformin which stimulates FGF21 in human liver cells (requires a doctor's prescription). Physical exercise has also been shown to increase FGF21 in young women.

FIVE

FGF21 AND LATE ADAPTIVE RESPONSE TO STARVATION IN HUMANS

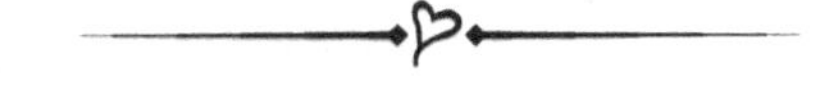

In mice, FGF21 is rapidly induced by fasting, mediates critical aspects of the adaptive starvation response, and displays a number of positive metabolic properties when administered pharmacologically.

In humans, however, fasting does not consistently increase FGF21, suggesting a possible evolutionary divergence in FGF21 function. Moreover, many key aspects of FGF21 function in mice have been identified in the context of transgenic overexpression or administration of supraphysiologic doses, rather than in a physiologic setting.

Here, we explored the dynamics and function of FGF21 in human volunteers during a 10-day fast. Unlike mice, which show an increase in circulating FGF21 after only 6 hours, human subjects did not have a notable surge in FGF21 until 7 to 10 days of fasting.

Moreover, we determined that FGF21 induction was associated with decreased thermogenesis and adiponectin, an observation that directly contrasts with previous reports based on supraphysiologic dosing.

Additionally, FGF21 levels increased after ketone induction, demonstrating that endogenous FGF21 does not drive starvation-mediated ketogenesis in humans. Instead, a longitudinal analysis of biologically relevant variables identified serum transaminases — markers of tissue breakdown — as predictors of FGF21.

These data establish FGF21 as a fasting-induced hormone in humans and indicate that FGF21 contributes to the late stages of adaptive starvation, when it may regulate the utilization of fuel derived from tissue breakdown.

As periods of famine were an important aspect of the human evolutionary environment, the body's adaptive ability during periods of starvation was a key survival advantage. Fibroblast growth factor 21 (FGF21) has been described as a key liver-secreted hormonal mediator of the adaptive response to starvation, a finding primarily based on data generated from mouse models. Functions attributed to FGF21 during starvation include driving

1. ketogenesis,
2. gluconeogenesis,
3. growth hormone resistance which prevents expenditure of energy on growth, and
4. disruption of the hypothalamic-pituitary-ovarian axis which minimizes the expenditure of energy on reproduction.

It might seem counterintuitive that a starvation-induced hormone would also prevent diet-induced obesity and improve glucose tolerance, but treatment of ob/ob mice with pharmacologic doses of FGF21 lowers glucose and insulin levels during oral glucose tolerance testing.

Furthermore, FGF21 transgenic mice demonstrate improved glucose clearance and insulin sensitivity as compared with their WT littermates. FGF21 mediates this improvement in glucose clearance in part through an insulin-independent pathway involving glucose transporter 1 (GLUT1).

FGF21 transgenic mice are also resistant to a high-fat/high-carbohydrate diet; despite eating more food than do their WT littermates, they gain less weight, an effect that appears to be at least partially mediated by induction of thermogenesis. Why a hormone that is upregulated during starvation would enhance weight loss and induce thermogenesis is unknown.

The confluence of positive preclinical data showing beneficial metabolic effects of FGF21 in mouse models has provided a rationale to develop FGF21 or related mimetics for the treatment of human obesity and diabetes mellitus despite ongoing ?uestions regarding the conservation of FGF21 regulation and function between mice and humans.

Indeed, the original paradigm of FGF21 as a fasting-induced hormone has not seamlessly translated to humans. One small study that measured serum FGF21 before and after a 7-day fast in patients with rheumatoid arthritis demonstrated a modest 74% increase in FGF21 levels. Subse?uently, however, numerous studies have demonstrated no change in FGF21 levels with fasting for up to 72 hours.

Moreover, women with anorexia nervosa, a state of chronic nutritional deprivation, have reduced or similar levels of FGF21 as compared with levels in normal-weight controls.

Therefore, it is unknown whether these contradictory results are due to interstudy differences in the duration of fasting or whether they speak to a lack of generalizability of the fasting effect observed in rheumatoid arthritis.

Therefore, the primary aim of this study was to test the hypothesis that fasting induces circulating levels of FGF21 in humans and, secondarily, to determine whether the functions attributed to FGF21 in murine models also apply to humans.

We reasoned that a prolonged fast was necessary to definitively test this hypothesis and therefore recruited healthy individuals to undergo a medically supervised fast for 10 days, following a previously published protocol. We performed;

- serial measurements of circulating FGF21 levels and factors that have been functionally linked to FGF21 in animal models, such as ketones;
- pre- and post-fasting PET/MRI scans to measure brown adipose tissue (BAT); and
- serial transcriptional analysis of white adipose tissue (WAT) biopsy specimens to assess the expression of FGF21 pathway genes. The analyses of multiple time points over the course of the 10-day fast allowed us to leverage a relatively small cohort to dissect both the fasting-mediated dynamics of FGF21 and to gain a greater understanding of the role of FGF21 in the adaptive starvation response.

SIX

FGF21 AND LATE ADAPTIVE RESPONSE TO STARVATION IN HUMANS

In mice, FGF21 is rapidly induced by fasting, mediates critical aspects of the adaptive starvation response, and displays a number of positive metabolic properties when administered pharmacologically.

In humans, however, fasting does not consistently increase FGF21, suggesting a possible evolutionary divergence in FGF21 function. Moreover, many key aspects of FGF21 function in mice have been identified in the context of transgenic overexpression or administration of supraphysiologic doses, rather than in a physiologic setting.

Here, we explored the dynamics and function of FGF21 in human volunteers during a 10-day fast. Unlike mice, which show an increase in circulating FGF21 after only 6 hours, human subjects did not have a notable surge in FGF21 until 7 to 10 days of fasting.

Moreover, we determined that FGF21 induction was associated with decreased thermogenesis and adiponectin, an observation that directly contrasts with previous reports based on supraphysiologic dosing.

Additionally, FGF21 levels increased after ketone induction, demonstrating that endogenous FGF21 does not drive starvation-mediated ketogenesis in humans. Instead, a longitudinal analysis of biologically relevant variables identified serum transaminases — markers of tissue breakdown — as predictors of FGF21.

These data establish FGF21 as a fasting-induced hormone in humans and indicate that FGF21 contributes to the late stages of adaptive starvation, when it may regulate the utilization of fuel derived from tissue breakdown.

As periods of famine were an important aspect of the human evolutionary environment, the body's adaptive ability during periods of starvation was a key survival advantage. Fibroblast growth factor 21 (FGF21) has been described as a key liver-secreted hormonal mediator of the adaptive response to starvation, a finding primarily based on data generated from mouse models. Functions attributed to FGF21 during starvation include driving

1. ketogenesis,
2. gluconeogenesis,
3. growth hormone resistance which prevents expenditure of energy on growth, and
4. disruption of the hypothalamic-pituitary-ovarian axis which minimizes the expenditure of energy on reproduction.

It might seem counterintuitive that a starvation-induced hormone would also prevent diet-induced obesity and improve glucose tolerance, but treatment of ob/ob mice with pharmacologic doses of FGF21 lowers glucose and insulin levels during oral glucose tolerance testing.

Furthermore, FGF21 transgenic mice demonstrate improved glucose clearance and insulin sensitivity as compared with their WT littermates. FGF21 mediates this improvement in glucose clearance in part through an insulin-independent pathway involving glucose transporter 1 (GLUT1).

FGF21 transgenic mice are also resistant to a high-fat/high-carbohydrate diet; despite eating more food than do their WT littermates, they gain less weight, an effect that appears to be at least partially mediated by induction of thermogenesis. Why a hormone that is upregulated during starvation would enhance weight loss and induce thermogenesis is unknown.

The confluence of positive preclinical data showing beneficial metabolic effects of FGF21 in mouse models has provided a rationale to develop FGF21 or related mimetics for the treatment of human obesity and diabetes mellitus despite ongoing ?uestions regarding the conservation of FGF21 regulation and function between mice and humans.

Indeed, the original paradigm of FGF21 as a fasting-induced hormone has not seamlessly translated to humans. One small study that measured serum FGF21 before and after a 7-day fast in patients with rheumatoid arthritis demonstrated a modest 74% increase in FGF21 levels. Subse?uently, however, numerous studies have demonstrated no change in FGF21 levels with fasting for up to 72 hours.

Moreover, women with anorexia nervosa, a state of chronic nutritional deprivation, have reduced or similar levels of FGF21 as compared with levels in normal-weight controls.

Therefore, it is unknown whether these contradictory results are due to interstudy differences in the duration of fasting or whether they speak to a lack of generalizability of the fasting effect observed in rheumatoid arthritis.

Therefore, the primary aim of this study was to test the hypothesis that fasting induces circulating levels of FGF21 in humans and, secondarily, to determine whether the functions attributed to FGF21 in murine models also apply to humans.

We reasoned that a prolonged fast was necessary to definitively test this hypothesis and therefore recruited healthy individuals to undergo a medically supervised fast for 10 days, following a previously published protocol. We performed;

- serial measurements of circulating FGF21 levels and factors that have been functionally linked to FGF21 in animal models, such as ketones;
- pre- and post-fasting PET/MRI scans to measure brown adipose tissue (BAT); and
- serial transcriptional analysis of white adipose tissue (WAT) biopsy specimens to assess the expression of FGF21 pathway genes. The analyses of multiple time points over the course of the 10-day fast allowed us to leverage a relatively small cohort to dissect both the fasting-mediated dynamics of FGF21 and to gain a greater understanding of the role of FGF21 in the adaptive starvation response.

SEVEN

FGF 21 AND FASTING

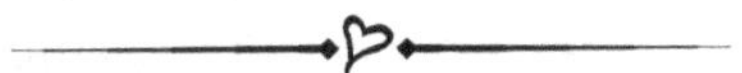

According to the NIH (2016), the protein encoded by FGF21 is part of the FGF (fibroblast growth factor) family. This family of proteins deals with tissue repair, cell growth, tumor growth, morphogenesis, and other processes.

Data from mouse models (FGF21 transgenic mice) attribute various functions to FGF21:

- induction of ketogenesis and gluconeogenesis
- growth hormone resistance (preventing energy expenditure on growth)
- disruption of the HPO axis (minimizing energy expenditure on reproduction)

Researchers explain;

FGF21 transgenic mice are also resistant to a high-fat/high-carbohydrate diet; despite eating more food than do their WT littermates, they gain less weight, an effect that appears to be at least partially mediated by induction of thermogenesis.

Why a hormone that is upregulated during starvation would enhance weight loss and induce thermogenesis is unknown.

They think that it is important to study the metabolic effects of FGF21 to determine how the mechanisms observed in mice apply to humans. If these mechanisms remain consistent, they would provide rationale for further developing FGF21 mimetics for treating diabetes and obesity.

Previous human studies, according to the researchers have not shown consistency in these mechanisms:

One small study that measured serum FGF21 before and after a 7-day fast in patients with rheumatoid arthritis demonstrated a modest 74% increase in FGF21 levels. Subse?uently, however, numerous studies have demonstrated no change in FGF21 levels with fasting for up to 72 hours. Moreover, women with anorexia nervosa, a state of chronic nutritional deprivation, have reduced or similar levels of FGF21 as compared with levels in normal-weight controls.

Thus, they wanted to test the hypothesis that fasting increases circulating levels of FGF21 and see if the mechanisms of actions of FGF21 observed in mice also apply to humans.

EIGHT
CONCLUSION

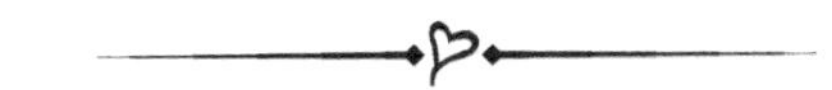

Researchers around the world are lauding the discovery of a 'miracle hormone' that seems to be able to get your metabolism in order, perk up your immune system and maybe even help you live longer.

Called Fibroblast growth factor 21 (FGF21), researchers at University of Sydney's Charles Perkins Centre say they've found a diet that boosts FGF21 levels — in mice — and are optimistic the findings will translate to humans. These findings rethink the strategic balance of carbohydrates and proteins in a healthy diet — again.

Fibroblast growth factor 21 (FGF21) is the first known endocrine signal activated by protein restriction. Although FGF21 is robustly elevated in low-protein environments, increased FGF21 is also seen in various other contexts such as fasting, overfeeding, ketogenic diets, and high-carbohydrate diets, leaving its nutritional context and physiological role unresolved and controversial.

9 781639 202164